The Benefits of Exercise for Smokers

And how exercise may help you quit smoking faster!

Dr. OneHeart

Introduction

Did you know that though smoking increases the risk of dying from heart problems and respiratory diseases that practicing regular physical exercise can reduce that risk?

Not only does exercise reduces the risk of dying from smoking, but it also improves the quality of life of the smoker since they tend to suffer from less medical problems and diseases known to be associated with smoking.

Quality of life speaks to the level of satisfaction a person is able to enjoy in their daily life, despite their financial circumstances.

A person who is trying to quit smoking can also find a trusted partner in exercising, as the chemical changes it produce in the body will definitely make the goal easier to accomplish.

However, not every smoker is recommended to do regular exercise. The type of exercise and the most suitable schedule to follow are also things to be taken into consideration.

This booklet aims to walk you through the many benefits of exercise for smokers, including if you are trying to quit smoking; the best types of exercises that may benefit you, when to practice these exercises, how frequently you should do these exercises, who should avoid doing them and so much more.

Table of Contents

The Effects of smoking on the body

As I am sure you already know, smoking has many harmful effects on the body, hence why there are millions of campaigns yearly to try and get people to quit smoking and ban Tobacco use.

If you didn't know most cigarettes contain Tobacco which when burn releases many substances into the air (over 7000), at least 250 of these substances are known to be toxic and around 70 are known to cause cancer. The smoker or those around them then inhale the smoke containing these toxic chemicals which can result in many harmful effects and diseases in the body.

The main substance that is released and causes addiction however, is nicotine.

Nicotine is naturally present in tobacco though some companies may add extra nicotine to their products.

The definition of smoking, which is the inhalation of smoke from the burning of cigarettes or tobacco, does not technically include vaping, since vaping is described as the inhalation of vapours from e-cigarettes.

While vaping is usually described as a safer alternative to smoking, the jury is still out on that one, as e-cigarettes also contain their own toxic chemicals, though these may be significantly less than those contained in traditional cigarettes.

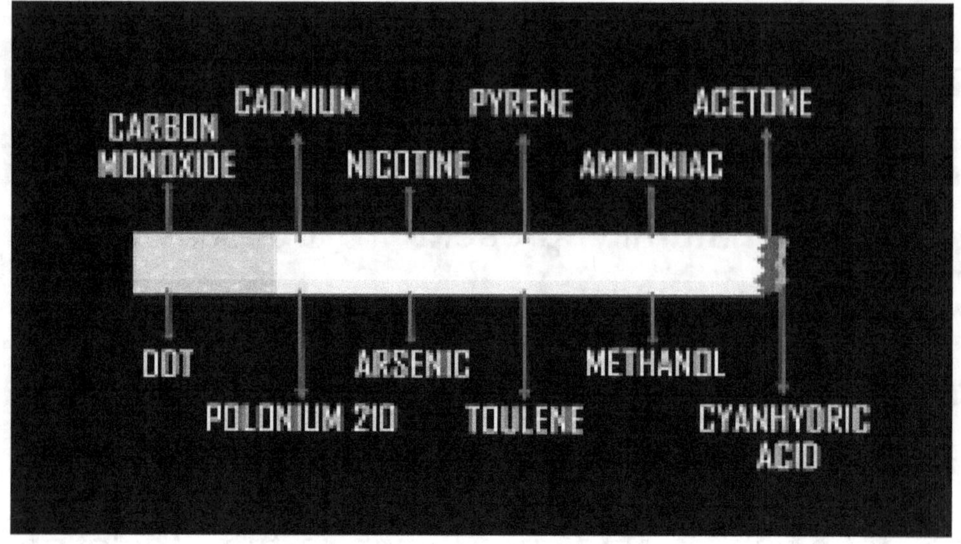

Two of the most harmful substances that are released from cigarette smoking are tar and carbon monoxide.

Tar is a known cancerogenic substance that means it is known to cause cancer.

Carbon monoxide decreases the amount of oxygen in our body: one of the reasons why smoking is said to affect or cause damage to every single organ in our bodies (since all body organs rely on oxygen to function properly.)

Based on the statistics it is reported that a smoker is three times more likely to die than a person who has never smoked. Among the highest causes of deaths in smokers are heart attack, cancer, stroke and lung diseases. But smoking is responsible for many other diseases and can also cause infertility and miscarriages in women.

Smoking is also reported to be the second leading risk factor for deaths worldwide, behind hypertension or high blood pressure, killing about 8 million people worldwide yearly.

Smoking is a Disease:

This is because based on the definition of the World Health Organization's (WHO) definition of Disease, which considers that once there is a rupture in the well-being or health of the person, even if there is no actual disease then it still classifies as such.

It is also considered to be the principal preventable epidemic that is still plaguing public health officials. Though smoking is avoidable it still continues to be widespread all across the world because the health effects appears years or even decades after continuous use; plus cigarettes are cheap and heavily promoted by cigarette companies.

When a person smokes it can leave them feeling more relaxed, optimistic and happy. Within the first 24 hours after smoking the person can start to develop nicotine withdrawal symptoms which motivates them to start smoking again, overtime however, an habitual smoker will develop certain signs and symptoms of smoking:

Signs and symptoms of a Habitual Smoker:

- Feeling tired or lack of energy (this may improve after smoking)

- Lack of appetite (which usually increases after smoking)

- Yellowing of the teeth

- Hoarseness due to smoking

- Cough during the mornings

- Diffuse chest pains

- Shortness of breath or difficulty breathing after prolonged use

- Impotence or decrease (libido) in the desire to have sex

➡ May suffer from bronquitis from time to time

Some diseases that may be more frequent in smokers:

➡ High blood pressure

➡ Heart diseases

➡ Stroke

➡ Chronic Obstructive Pulmonary Disease (COPD)- long term coughing and shortness of breath

➡ Lung cancer

➡ Other Cancers, such as mouth and throat cancers

➡ Diabetes

➡ Eye diseases, such as cataracts (Cloudy or

blurry visions)

➡ Tuberculosis

➡ Airway infections

➡ Digestive Diseases such as stomach ulcers

➡ Problems with the immune system (system

that fights off diseases in the body)

➡ Rheumatoid Arthritis

➡ Infertility and miscarriages in women

It is also reported that women who smokes and

take birth control pills are 39 times more likely to

suffer a heart attack than women who do not smoke.

Smoking also reduces vitamin C concentrations in the body which can make it difficult for cuts to heal.

Most of the harmful effects of smoking are seen over a long period of time; reason why smoking continues to be a preventable epidemic that is really hard to get rid of.

How exercise can lead to a better quality of life for a smoker

Quality of life according to the Merriam Webster's dictionary is the degree to which a person or group is healthy, comfortable and able to enjoy the activities of daily living. There is no doubt therefore that our health plays a very important role in how we view our life and the satisfaction we draw from it.

The difference between a smoker and a non-smoker is that a person who smokes is prone to so much more health hazards when compared to their counter-parts.

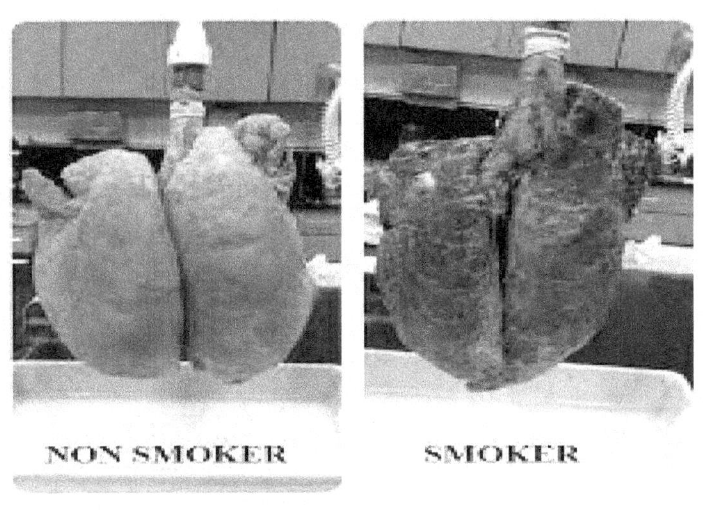

Lungs of a smoker compared to a non-smoker

Because the concept of quality of life is so diverse and subjective, a person who smokes can still consider their quality of life to be better than a person who does not smoke based on the degree of satisfaction they feel with their own lives. However in terms of health, it is fair to conclude that a person who does not smoke would enjoy a better quality of life than a smoker because of all the health benefits associated with not smoking.

And while the above may be true, it is also fair to conclude that a smoker who participates in regular physical activities would also enjoy a better quality of life than a smoker who does not; this due to the many benefits of exercise for the body in general.

✓ **So in conclusion a smoker who exercises is expected to have a better quality of life than a smoker who does not; but all in all the best quality of life (in terms of health) belong to non-smokers!**

Heavy smokers or people who smoke on the daily have higher risks of suffering from multiple health issues and poorer quality of life.

While they may avoid nicotine withdrawal symptoms and may feel relaxed and satisfied each time they smoke, in the long run the continuous and prolonged use of tobacco will inevitably result in damages to their health and negative changes in their lifestyle.

Cardiovascular, respiratory, digestive diseases or a combination of these once developed for example, can result in continuous absence from school or work which can cause the person to lose their job and start affecting the quality of their performance and education etc.

These diseases may also start to limit a person's ability to participate in normal day to day activities when they do not have the physical strength and stamina to do what they used to do; Treatment and medications for heart diseases, cancer, stroke or other diseases in general are not cheap; plus it is very expensive for people who are bed ridden to pay to take care of their health and other expenses.

These are just some of the ways poor health can result in poorer quality of life for smokers. Not only does smoking have the potential to make you sick and drain your finances, but the physical, emotional, psychological and social stresses added unto it, can't help but to start affecting the way a person will start to view and appreciate their life.

And while smokers are at a greater risk of suffering from poorer quality of life, there is still hope of improving that quality of life through exercise.

While admittedly exercise is not a panacea for the health hazards of smoking, it can definitely improve a smokers health risks:
Studies have shown that exercises not only reduce a person's risk of dying from certain diseases, such as heart diseases and cancer, but that it may also prevent the smoker from developing them in the first place.

Improvement in health due to exercise, should also result in an improvement in the quality of life of a smoker.

Now let's look at how exercise can result in a better quality of life for smokers in more details, by focusing on the many health benefits it offers for this group.

The benefits of exercise for Smokers

Exercise in smokers does not only improve mortality rates but also morbidity rates. This means that a person who smokes and does regular exercise is not only less likely to die from certain diseases such as heart attacks and strokes, but also that they are less likely to develop them in the first place.

Apart from the improvements it causes in death and disease rates, exercise also adds the extra benefit of reducing a person's desire to smoke making them more likely to quit.

While exercise is not an excuse to not quit smoking since not smoking is the healthiest alternative, for chronic smokers or for people who have not been able to kick the habit, exercise is definitely the healthier choice for them compared to a sedentary (not physically active) lifestyle.

<u>Now let's take a look at the statistics:</u>

1) Investigations have shown that smokers who exercise reduce their risk of having cardiovascular (heart and blood vessels) diseases by 35% and lung cancer by 74%.

2) Dr. Judith Garcia-Aymerich (of Medical Investigations in Spain), have reported that smokers who are moderately to very active will reduce their risk of getting any lung disease by 20 %. Also that by sticking to a regular cardiovascular training regimen three times per week will reduce the risk of dying from heart attacks and strokes by 40 %.

3) Exercise also reduces the risk of fatality (or deaths) by reducing the chances of dying from heart attacks, strokes, cancer and diabetes (sugar) by 30-40%.

4) The risk of dying from cancer goes down by 25% compared to smokers who are not physically active.

*It is reported that pregnant women are also more likely to quit smoking if they participate in physical exercises and maintain a regular schedule.

Now we know some of the statistics of how exercise may mitigate or lessen mortality and morbidity rates in smokers, let's also take a further look at how smoking cause a protective effect in the body of smokers who exercise compared to those who do not.

Protective effects of exercise <u>on the heart and blood vessels:</u>

- One of the main systems of the body that smoking affects severely is the cardiovascular system. Increase heart rates, hardening of the blood vessels, being more prone to blood clots and heart attacks are just a few of the harmful effects of smoking.

  Exercise however will have the opposite effect since it is known to improve cardiovascular functions and causes an increase in HDL cholesterol (the good cholesterol) in the body.

  This type of cholesterol removes other forms of cholesterol or fats from your bloodstream, therefore making you less prone to suffer from atherosclerosis (narrowing and hardening of the blood vessels) and heart diseases.

So a smoker who does exercises in a sense is fighting back the harmful effects that smoking is causing on the heart and blood vessels and while it may not be the perfect situation, a smoker who gives their body the opportunity to fight back is still at a better advantage than one who does not.

Protective effects of exercise on the lungs and airways:

The fact that when you smoke you are breathing in hundreds of toxic chemicals in the body means that the respiratory system is the main system affected.

Airway and lung inflammation not only cause narrowing of the airways, but also cause less oxygen to pass through the lungs to other organs in the body. Carbon monoxide and tar build up in the lungs will also worsen the amount of oxygen in the body.

So it is a double edge sword when it comes to exercise and smoking; for not only does exercise improve lung function and the amount of oxygen in the body, but too smokers already have less oxygen in their body compared to non-smokers. This will undoubtedly affect their ability to do exercise in the first place, since muscles need oxygen to perform properly.

A smoker who exercises therefore may feel weak and less energetic or become breathless and tired a whole lot quicker compared to a non-smoker.

Therefore it is definitely harder for smokers to keep up regular physical activities, but if they make the effort and continue, then not only will it build up their physical endurance overtime but it will also decrease their chances of suffering and dying from lung cancer and other lung diseases in the end.

Studies have shown that once you lose lung functions from smoking, even if you quit you don't really gain them back. However, exercise will improve your lung capacity and

boost your fitness, so you suffer from less breathlessness and won't get tired as quickly.

Protective effects of exercise on the brain and mental functions:

- Atherosclerosis, reduced blood flow and low oxygen concentration that occur as a result of smoking can have very deleterious effects on a person's brain. Stroke is frequent in smokers, but there are also the mental and psychological effects also left to consider. Nicotine addiction and nicotine withdrawal symptoms may result in anxiety, depression and irritability when a person stays too long without smoking.

  Cognitive decline in smokers tend to develop faster than in non- smokers and the statistics is even worse for men than in women; based on a 2015 research review smokers are 30% more likely to suffer from dementia.

Exercise and in particular aerobic exercise offers protection to the brain against Dementia and Alzheimer's diseases. Cognitive functions such as memory and thinking are also better in people who are physically active.

The risk of stroke is significantly decreased due to exercise because exercise improve your cardiovascular health and allows for improve blood flow to the brain, but it also reduces stress and inflammation in general which are also risk factors for stroke.

Protective effects of exercise against cancers:

- There are many substances in cigarette smoke that not only make you prone to developing lung cancer, but also cancer anywhere else in the body for example. It is reported that 9 out of 10 lung cancer deaths are caused by direct smoking or second-hand smoking. Mouth and throat cancer, laryngeal or voice-box cancer, oesophageal, kidney and bladder cancers are just a few examples of other cancers cigarette smokers are prone to.

Did you know that men who smoke are more likely to die from prostate cancers than men who have the disease but do not smoke? Research has shown that exercise reduce the chances of developing cancer, but it also does more than that; it also decrease the chances of cancer relapse after treatment and the survival rate for cancer is better in people who do exercises.

Protective effects of exercise <u>for the digestive system</u>:

- Smoking can cause many digestive diseases, such as Crohn's disease, gallstones, Gastroesophageal Reflux Disease (GERD) which causes heart burns and peptic ulcer disease.

Peptic ulcers are sores in the lining of your stomach or the beginning of the small intestines, caused by stomach acids and are usually very painful.

Exercise can help these ulcers heal faster for several reasons: increased blood flow to the stomach, along with higher amounts of oxygen and less inflammation to the area will definitely cause cuts to heal more rapidly.

Gut and intestinal activity are also improved from doing exercises, making them work more quickly and efficiently.

Heartburns may improve because stomach acid drains faster.

Exercise also helps to prevent the formation of gallstones since these tend to form more in people who are overweight, and exercise causes you to lose weight and also reduce fats in the bloodstream.

Protective effects of Exercise on the Immune System:

- Not only do you breathe in many toxic substances from cigarette smoke which leaves you susceptible to developing so many diseases, but the fact that smoking impairs your immune system also means that it limits the body's potential to fight off these diseases as well.

  Exercise however, improve immune functions and therefore will also reduce the rates of cancer and infections in smokers.

  Smokers tend to suffer more frequently from acute and chronic bronchitis (Inflammation of the airways) and COPD, but increased exercise that boosts your immune system and make antibodies stronger will reduce the likelihood of contracting these diseases or at least reduce the amount of time you suffer from them.

Protective effects **against Diabetes and Rheumatoid Arthritis:**

Smoking also increases your risk of other diseases such as Diabetes and Rheumatoid Arthritis.

Exercise is known to reduce glucose levels in the blood and at the same time increase insulin sensitivity of the cells in the body, which means it can prevent type 2 diabetes or delay its development.

It may also help with preventing long- term complications of diabetes, such as heart problems.

Smoking does not only cause inflammation in the lungs, but also in other areas of the body, such as bones and joints.

The pain associated with Rheumatoid Arthritis (RA) is worse in people who smoke, studies have shown.

They also tend to have more joint damage and remission is less likely.

Exercise has so many contradictory effects to smoking in arthritic patients.

It is known to reduce joint pain and stiffness, increase flexibility and improve muscle and joint strength amongst other things. These improve the smoker's chances of remission and may slow down the progression of joint damage.

<u>To summarize:</u>

Exercise holds many benefits for everyone in general and not just smokers.

Persons who participate in regular physical exercise and have an active lifestyle are healthier than persons who are sedentary.

In smokers this is no different: smokers who have active lifestyles have more health benefits compared to smokers who do not exercise.

Exercise will oppose many of the harmful effects of smoking, and in many cases will either eliminate them completely or reduce their severity, making it a very suitable recommendation for smokers who haven't been able to quit or are trying to quit.

Smokers who do regular exercise usually benefit from a better quality of life than smokers who are sedentary.

Exercise reduces morbidity and mortality rates in smokers, which means there is a lower probability of suffering from certain medical conditions and even death.

Besides, reduction in morbidity and mortality rates means that smokers who do regular exercise also have higher life- expectancy -that is they tend to live longer than sedentary smokers.

Based on a study done in 2018, smokers who are physically active increase their life- expectancy by 3.7 years. Smokers who quitted and stayed active increased their life- expectancy by 5.6 years.

Apart from all those benefits, smokers who exercise are more likely to quit smoking and have lower relapse rates compared to smokers who are sedentary.

Let's take a deeper look into why exercise can help you quit smoking.

How exercise influence smoking cessation

There are several reasons why exercise may help you quit smoking faster.

Reason No. 1

Exercise can decrease a person's cravings for nicotine and therefore for smoking

Nicotine produces chemical changes in the brain of a smoker, which makes them dependent or addicted to it.

When a person smokes the nicotine stimulates the pleasure centres in the brain, at first the smoker will feel more relaxed, have better concentration and experience less anxiety, stress and appetite. Once the nicotine effect starts to wear off the person begins to experience withdrawal symptoms, such as headaches, anxiety, breathlessness, irritability, nausea, anger etc. These symptoms will influence the smoker to smoke again to try and curb the symptoms. Every time this cycle repeats the smoker becomes more and more dependent on smoking.

One of the theories as to why exercise reduces the cravings for nicotine and smoking is that when we exercise our body releases dopamine (a chemical substance responsible for pleasure). This dopamine then competes with the nicotine in the pleasure centres of our brain, which means it decreases the amount of nicotine acting on our brain, but at the same time gives the same amount of pleasure and relaxation that a person feels right after smoking.

The continuous reduction of nicotine means that in time there will be a regression of the chemical changes in the brain that was caused by smoking.

The less you smoke the more desensitized the brain becomes to the nicotine.

Overtime the cravings will decrease or be less intense, until eventually they will fade away completely.

Did you know?

Did you know that when you smoke it causes changes in your brain? This is due to the high concentrations of nicotine.

A person who smokes has higher levels of nicotinic receptors in their brain than non-smokers. An Addicted person may have billions of nicotinic receptors compared to non-smokers, since each time a person smoke these numbers tend to increase.

When you quit smoking, the number of these receptors starts to decrease until eventually they return to normal levels.

When this happens you crave smoking less, but also the intensity of the cravings will decrease until eventually they disappear completely.

<h1 style="text-align:center">Reason No.2</h1>

A person who is trying to quit smoking will experience nicotine withdrawal symptoms, within the first 24 hours, these symptoms tend to be worse around day 3 or 4 after quitting. Nicotine withdrawal symptoms include: headaches, nausea, difficulty concentrating, anxiety, irritability, mood swings and anger, intense cravings for cigarettes and sleep disorders amongst other things. It is not life threatening, unless there is some complication.

The severity of these symptoms can hinder a person's chances of quitting due to the intense cravings for cigarettes to relieve the symptoms. Studies have shown that exercise does cause a reduction in the intensity of these symptoms and if the smoker is able to keep up with an exercise regimen they will be more likely to quit. Also withdrawal syndrome may come with difficulty to sleep in some individuals, which exercise may also improve making it easier to quit.

<u>Reason No.3</u>

<u>Exercise reduce stress which may be one of the reason for smoking in the first place-</u>

Studies have shown that exercise distracts from stressful thoughts and emotions, resulting in less anxiety and depression.

Because stress have been inculpated as a reason why many persons turn to smoking, less stress, anxiety and depression should make it easier for them to cope and facilitate quitting.

Studies show that people who are depressed are twice as likely to smoke compared to people who are not depressed.

If you think that stress is one of the reasons why you smoke, try sticking to a regular exercise schedule and see if this decrease your desire to smoke or reduce the amount of cigarettes you smoke daily.

Did you know?

Did you know that though smoking causes an immediate sense of relaxation it does not really get rid of anxiety or depression; in fact it may increase it due to nicotine withdrawal symptoms; because the reason why you turn to smoking is still not dealt with.

Reason No. 4

Exercise makes you lose weight and so reduce the anxiety of gaining weight when trying to quit;

Some smokers are reluctant to stop smoking because they are afraid they may start gaining weight.

Smoking reduces a person's appetite and speeds up their metabolism meaning calories burn faster, making it harder for them to gain weight.

Some people who are trying to quit therefore starts to gain weight; if they view this as a problem they may be hesitant to quit smoking.

Not only does exercise cause you to lose weight, but it also holds so many other health benefits for you-

So if your anxiety comes from the fear of gaining weight when you are trying to quit, then try participating in regular physical exercise;
Not only should that reduce your anxiety, but also improve your overall mood and health all the while reducing your cravings for smoking in the process. You could also try changing your diet along with doing regular exercise to also help you lose weight.

- ✓ Also doing exercise might be a good distraction to take your mind off smoking: like substituting a good habit for a bad one!

- ✓ People who have already quit smoking and are physically active tend to have lower relapse rates than smokers who quit and do not continue to do regular exercises.

Exercises for smokers

Smokers tend to be less fit than non-smokers. When they participate in physical activities they have less endurance: they become tired and breathless a whole lot faster and they also have poorer performance doing exercises. Injuries from exercises are also more frequent in smokers.

Despite all these limitations, exercise holds so many benefits and improvements for the health of smokers that not doing them would be an oversight.

The benefits of exercise extends to all group of smokers, whether casual or chronic smokers, or those who are trying to quit.

While smoking alters the chemical structure of the brain causing addiction, exercise also cause many chemical changes in the body resulting in many positive effects, one of which is to reduce the exposition of the body to the harmful effects of smoking.

Aerobic Exercise

Aerobic exercise is the best exercise recommended for smokers and is a type of cardiovascular conditioning.

The term aerobic means "with oxygen."

This means that during aerobic exercise oxygen is being used to provide the energy your muscles need.

To do this it is important to control your breathing, but also the rate at which that energy is being produced.

That is why aerobic exercises tend to be less intense but of a longer duration compared to anaerobic respiration (which is the opposite).

There are many benefits of aerobic exercises. Not only does it better cardiovascular functions by strengthening heart muscles, reducing the heart rate at rest and lowering blood pressure; but it also improve lung functions, boosts your mood, activates the immune system, stimulate bone growth, improve mental health and reduce fatigue during exercise amongst many other things.

Due to the benefits mentioned above is why this kind of exercise is a very suitable choice for opposing the negative effects of smoking, since smoking cause many of the opposite effects that these exercise are known to improve.

Aerobic Exercise also reduces the risk of heart disease, Type 2 Diabetes and stroke.

Deaths due to cardiovascular diseases are also less frequent.

Aerobic exercise however, is not the best for building muscles or burning fats.

That is why smokers who are afraid of gaining weight when they are trying to quit, should try adding some amount of anaerobic exercise to their aerobics schedule, as anaerobic exercise are more intense and better for fat burning and weight loss.

Usually to maintain a regular routine, exercise should be done at least three times per week for no less than 30 mins. each time.

Here is a list of Aerobic Exercise you can try doing:

- Walking

- Running (distance running)

- Riding a bicycle

- Swimming

- Skipping or jump rope

- Jogging

- Skateboarding

- Climbing stairs

- Kick- boxing

- Doing jumping jacks

➡ You can also try rowing and skiing

➡ Or other indoor activities such as:

✓ Step aerobics
✓ Aerobic dancing, such as Zumba
✓ Using a treadmill
✓ Using an elliptical trainer

Try using a combination of these on a weekly basis to add diversity and flexibility to your schedule. This may make it more interesting and motivate you better to actually keep doing it.

It is also better if you plan ahead and write down your exercise schedule, so you can look at it over and over again making it easier to memorize.

Also don't make a schedule that is too heavy that you know you won't stick to or have the time and energy to maintain.

It is best to start out small and then progressively increase in time and intensity.

Other Exercises for Smokers

Anaerobic Exercises

- While Aerobic exercise is the best exercise for smokers, it is not the only exercise that can be done. As stated above smokers who are trying to quit and are afraid of gaining weight or smokers who just want to lose weight in general, should try combining both aerobic and anaerobic exercise weekly, since aerobic exercise alone is not optimal for weight loss.

  Examples of Anaerobic exercises to consider are:

  ✓ Sprints or short distance running

- Doing circuit exercises (repeating a series of the same exercise within the time frame), such as push-ups, jumping jacks, jump squats and mountain climbers etc.

- Strength training

<u>Isometric Exercises</u>

- Also apart from aerobic exercise, maybe you could try doing isometric exercises since these exercises have the potential to immediately reduce the desire to smoke.

  When you are having intense cravings these exercise may help by providing immediate relief.

  In isometric exercise the person is static or not moving.

  Examples of these exercises include planking, where the person holds a particular pose for a period of time. Also wall sits and certain yoga poses such as tree pose etc.

Deep- Breathing Exercises

- The benefits of deep- breathing exercise are still being investigated for use in smokers.

  These exercises may improve lung capacity and may also be a form of replacement therapy for the satisfaction of the deep inhalation of cigarette smoke that persons who are trying to quit or have already quit may crave.

  It is also said to improve the cravings for smoking making it easier to quit.

<u>Mental Exercises</u>

- Apart from physical Exercise, mental exercise can improve brain functions in smokers as well.

Engaging in mentally stimulating activities can build cognitive functions such as memory and thinking and can delay the onset of Dementia and Alzheimer in smokers.

Examples of mentally stimulating activities you can try are:

- ✓ Reading books,

- ✓ Learning a new language

- ✓ Try solving math problems or puzzles

- ✓ Learn a new skill

- ✓ Stay socially active engaging and communicating more with friends and family etc.

<u>Other things to know:</u>

- Persons who suffer from a compulsive desire to smoke when faced with certain triggers that may influence their desire for a cigarette, such as seeing somebody light a cigarette, feeling restless or smelling cigarette smoke for example, can benefit from doing exercises in these situations as well.

  When faced with the trigger instead of smoking try doing a short exercise session as a substitution method for smoking.

The duration, frequency and intensity of Exercise in smokers

To stay physically active exercise should be practiced routinely or on a regular basis. It is recommended therefore, to practice exercises for at least 3 times per week for 30 minutes each time.

Warm up exercises should be done for 5 minutes, followed by 30-40 minutes of aerobic exercises and then 5 minutes of cooling-down exercises.

Warm- up exercises free up your joints and muscles making you less prone to getting joint and muscle damage during exercise.

They also increase blood flow to your muscles and prepare them for more strenuous exercise.

Examples of these include stretching your hamstrings, jumping jacks, leg or arm circles and squats.

Cooling down exercises help your heart rate and temperature to gradually return to normal and allow your muscles to stretch, making you feel more relaxed after exercising. Exercises such as walking or stretching are examples of these.

Though smokers can see result with doing less exercise than with what is stated here, sticking to this regimen is usually the best to see satisfactory results.

Smokers who are just beginning to do exercise can start with once or twice a week and slowly progress from there, since that may be more realistic for them.

Some smokers will find it harder to be motivated to do regular exercise than others and that is why everybody will need to find their own method that works best for them. For example, a person can choose to start off by doing exercise for 20 mins. each day and the progressively increase from 20 mins. up to an hour daily, depending on their schedule, preference and motivation.

Intensity of exercise means how hard you are working and can be monitored by your heart rate.

Different smokers will have different limitations to the intensity of exercise they can manage based on their fitness level.

Aerobic exercises which are recommended for smokers are usually low to moderate intensity.
This may make it more realistic and manageable for smokers, especially those who are beginners or older, since smoking already reduces a person's capacity to do and maintain physical activities.

Low to moderate intensity over longer periods of time means a person has a better chance of slowly building their strength and stamina.

Also studies have shown that exercises that are of a lower intensity, such as aerobic exercises are better to combat nicotine withdrawal symptoms than high intensity exercises, such as anaerobic exercises.

Precautions to take before doing these exercises:

- Usually it is recommended to not do exercises right after smoking, because the levels of carbon monoxide in the blood tends to be higher, which means oxygen concentrations are lower. Doing exercise will reduce oxygen concentrations even further which can affect your brain and muscles if severe.

- Smokers with COPD, that is chronic bronchitis and Emphysema, are not usually recommended to do exercise, because exercise will only increase the breathing difficulty they are already experiencing.

- Smokers with heart conditions, hypertension, diabetes, lung problems and arthritis may first need to speak to a doctor before starting an exercise program.

- Persons who develop certain signs and symptoms while exercising such as, chest pains or chest tightness, shortness of breath, dizziness, joint pain etc. may have other underlying health problems they are unaware of and should stop exercising right away and speak to their physician immediately.

Conclusion

Exercise has many unexpected benefits for smokers.

Smokers who exercise may suffer from fewer diseases and also have less chances of dying from many medical conditions such as heart attacks, strokes and cancers, compared to smokers who are sedentary.

Not only are morbidity and mortality rates improved in this group, but the quality of their lives tend to be better and they also benefit from increased life- expectancy.

Another important benefit is that smokers who exercise have a better advantage to quit smoking compared to those who do not do regular physical activity.

Exercise reduces a smoker's cravings for cigarettes and cause improvement in nicotine withdrawal symptoms.

Smokers who exercise may experience improvements in their mood, less stress and anxieties, making them feel better overall and also decrease their urge to smoke.

Smokers may experience some limitations when it comes to doing exercise when compared to non-smokers. They tend to become tired and breathless faster, sometimes just by doing normal day to day activities such as walking and climbing stairs and they are more prone to injuries due to exercise.

Aerobic exercise is the best exercise recommended for smokers and should be done on a regular basis, at least three times a week for 30 mins. However, everybody has to find a schedule that best works for them and also the type and intensity of the exercise they can manage.

Smokers who have other medical conditions such as COPD, Asthma, Hypertension (high blood pressure) and Diabetes should speak to their doctor before starting any exercise program.

Also if smokers experience certain symptoms such as chest pain and chest tightness, lightheadedness, shoulder pain etc. they should stop right away and contact their doctor.

All in all smokers who are physically active has many advantages due to exercise compared to smokers who do not.

Therefore though exercise is not a substitute for quitting smoking, it is a better option for smokers who are unable to quit, rather than a sedentary lifestyle.

Sources where information was obtained:

- http://americanheart.mediroom.com
- http://americanheart.org/presentar
- **Microsoft ® Encarta ® 2008. © 1993-2007 Microsoft Corporation.**
- **Advanced Biology for You. Gareth Williams.2000.**
- **World health organization (WHO)**
- **National Cancer Institute**
- **Lung Health Institute**
- **Mental Health foundation**
- **Center for Disease Control and Prevention (CDC)**
- **National Institute of Health**
- **Healthline**
- **Cleveland clinic**
- **John Hopkins Medicine**
- **Tobacco Induced Diseases (TID)**
- **Archivo de Bronconeumologia**
- **Mayoclinic**
- **Wikipedia**

Thank you for purchasing and Reading this E-book!

Blog: eyesthatseetutti.blogspot.com
Youtube: Dr.Oneheart